Heal Your Mind, Body, and Soul with Massage Therapy

KATHERINE E. SMITH, LMT

PAGE PUBLISHING, INC.
New York, NY

First originally published by Page Publishing, Inc. 2019

This publication is for informational purposes only and is not intended as medical advice. Medical advice should always be obtained from a qualified medical professional for any health conditions or symptoms associated with them. Every possible effort has been made in preparing and researching this material. We make no warranties with respect to the accuracy, applicability of its contents, or any omissions.

ISBN 978-1-64462-686-3 (Paperback)
ISBN 978-1-64462-687-0 (Digital)

Printed in the United States of America

To my husband, who encouraged me to write this book. Thank you for your love and support.

Contents

Introduction

What Is Massage Therapy?

Massage therapy is considered to be one of the oldest methods of healing, with the practice dating back to around 2000 BC.

The practice of massage therapy refers to the application of pres-

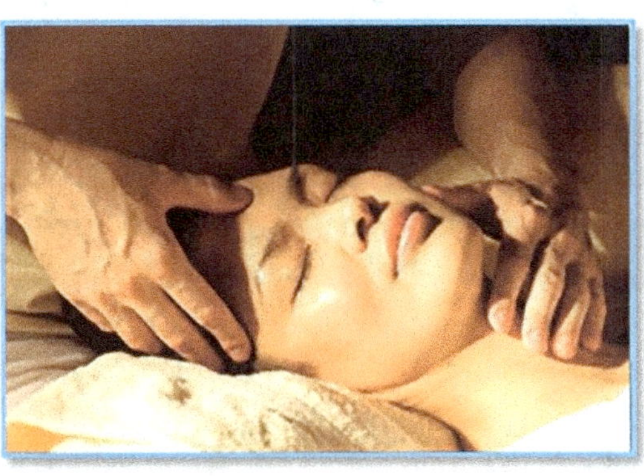

sure to the soft tissues of the body using different techniques such as friction, kneading, and vibration. This pressure is applied in order to manipulate the soft body tissues (muscles, ligaments, tendons, connective tissues), thus improving one's health and well-being.

There are many reasons to seek massage therapy. Some of the most notable health benefits of massages are the following:

- Reduced anxiety and stress
- Pain relief

- Improved strength of the immune system
- Relaxation of muscles
- Enhanced mood
- Improved heart health
- Enhanced blood flow
- Lower blood pressure
- Reduced risk of depression

Many professional and amateur athletes get regular massages to improve athletic performance and help with injury recovery.

According to the American Massage Therapy Association (AMTA), massage is a therapy that promotes complete and total wellness and health of both the mind and the body. According to an AMTA survey conducted in 2015, 88 percent of participants viewed massage as beneficial to overall health and wellness.

In modern times, massage is no longer a mere luxury but the most widely used type of alternative medicine therapy in hospitals for mental health, pain management, stress reduction, and general wellness. In fact, a lot of doctors are now prescribing massage therapy to their patients for pain and stress reduction. It used to be when a patient came in to see a doctor for pain and stress relief, doctors would prescribe painkillers and muscle relaxants.

However, a lot of people reported a lot of side effects from the medications which would be uncomfortable or even dangerous. So a lot of doctors have researched massage therapy through the years and have found out that massage therapy can reduce pain and stress without any side effects.

The popular forms of massage that can help with pain and stress reduction are the following:

- Swedish massage
- Deep-tissue massage
- Shiatsu massage
- Aromatherapy massage
- Hot-stone massage
- Reflexology massage

- Sports massage
- Lymph massage
- Healing touch / energy-healing massage
- Pregnancy massage
- Geriatric massage

Even though there are a lot of health benefits of massage, there are also contraindications and indications.

So what does contraindications mean? Contraindication is a term used to describe a situation where due to some physical issue, the client may have a negative reaction to the massage. For example, if a client had a fever, a massage would make the fever worse!

What does indications mean? Indications mean that a massage can be given to a client who would benefit from it in a positive way. For example, a client who has pain or muscle tension in their body would find relief after the massage.

Popular Forms of Massage

Swedish Massage

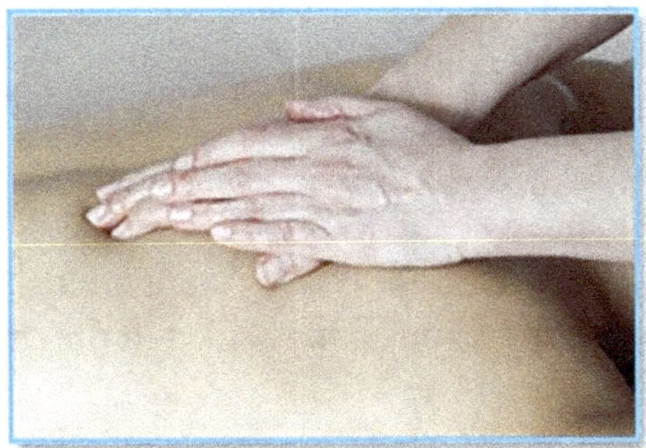

Swedish massage therapy is based around five different massage movements such as kneading movements, vibration, sliding movements, percussion, and rubbing.

What Is Swedish Massage?

A Swedish massage is a massage that includes both active and passive joint movements and stretching, with the assistance of a massage therapist, as well as a combination of kneading, vibration, percussion, rubbing, and sliding movements such as effleurage. Usually, the pressure for this type of massage is very light.

This type of massage helps improve blood circulation by having a positive effect on the soft tissues. Namely, good circulation will stimulate the body to clean and nourish soft tissues, such as the skin and muscles. Swedish massage is also known to significantly reduce stress, help heal injuries, and relieve pain.

Swedish massage is considered to be the foundation for many other types of massage therapies, including deep-tissue, sports, and aromatherapy massage methods.

History of Swedish Massage

So where did Swedish massage originate from? Swedish massage originated from Sweden in the 1700s by a man named Pehr Henrik Ling, who was born in 1776 in Smaaland, Sweden, and died in 1839. He was a Swedish physician and a fencing teacher. When he was younger, he served in the military and had suffered from rheumatism due to the bad weather conditions he faced in Europe.

Later on in his life, he found that the exercises and training through fencing helped reduce his pain. Plus he also incorporated gymnastics into his training. He was also very interested in the effects of passive and active stretching. This helped in the treatment for diseases and injuries.

Benefits of Swedish Massage

What are the benefits of Swedish massage? The benefits of Swedish massage include help with relaxation, relieve stress, heal scar tissue from injuries or surgeries, reduce and relieve pain, improve the immune system, reduce inflammation, increase blood flow, increase flexibility, reduce anxiety levels, and cleanse the body from impurities by stimulating lymph circulation for waste and toxic elimination.

Contraindications for Swedish Massage

What are the contraindications for a Swedish massage? The contraindications for a Swedish massage follow under three types of contraindications which are total, local, and medical.

Total means when a massage should not be performed at all! The total contraindications are the following:

- Fever

- Contagious diseases
- Cold or flu
- Under the influence of drugs or alcohol
- Prescription of pain medications
- Recent surgeries and acute injuries
- Neuritis
- Skin diseases

Local contraindications mean that the therapist can massage but not over any areas that are affected. Local contraindications are the following:

- Varicose veins
- Undiagnosed lumps or bumps
- Pregnancy
- Bruising
- Cuts
- Abrasions
- Sunburn
- Undiagnosed pain
- Inflammation, including arthritis

Medical contraindications mean that the massage can take place only if it has been approved in writing by a physician. Medical contraindications are the following:

- Cardiovascular conditions such as thrombosis, phlebitis, hypertension, and heart conditions
- Any condition already being treated by a medical practitioner
- Edema
- Psoriasis or eczema
- High blood pressure
- Osteoporosis
- Cancer
- Nervous or psychotic conditions

- Heart problems, angina and those with pacemakers
- Epilepsy
- Diabetes
- Bell's palsy, trapped or pinched nerves
- Gynecological infections

Deep-Tissue Massage

Although it's somewhat based on Swedish massage therapy, deep-tissue massage is different because it was designed to reach the deeper layers of the muscles and the connective tissues around them.

If you have ever taken part in a Swedish massage therapy, then deep-tissue massage might feel similar, mainly since the strokes are often the same or incredibly similar. The main difference is in the pressure being applied, where the therapist uses more pressure to apply deeper strokes to physically break down muscle adhesions that are the cause of the pain, inflammation, and limited range of motion. Muscle adhesions can also cause poor circulation.

What Is Deep-Tissue Massage?

Deep-tissue massage is a massage that uses firm pressure and slow strokes so the therapist can reach into the deeper layers of the muscles and the fascia, which is the connective tissue surrounding the muscles.

The most common strokes used in deep-tissue massage are stripping and friction. Stripping is when the therapist uses the elbow, forearm, knuckles, and thumbs to use deep, gliding pressure along the length of the muscle fibers. Friction is when the therapist applies pressure across the muscle to release adhesions and to help realign tissue fibers.

History of Deep-Tissue Massage

So where did deep-tissue massage originate from? Deep-tissue massage was originated by people who lived in the far east such as China, Korea, Japan, and India. It was also discovered by the ancient Greeks and the Egyptians.

Later in the 1800s, the deep-tissue techniques was first developed by Canadian physicians. One of the Canadian physicians was a woman by the name of Therese Pfrimmer. Therese Pfrimmer opened her first deep-tissue clinic in 1949. She also wrote a book in 1970 called *Muscles—Your Invisible Bonds*.

As time went on, deep-tissue massage gained popularity and is used today by practitioners to massage therapists and those who specialize in sports medicine and physical therapy.

Benefits of Deep-Tissue Massage

What are the benefits of deep-tissue massage? The benefits of deep-tissue massage are that it can help you heal from certain conditions such as lower-back pain and limited mobility and recover from injuries such as whiplash and falls, repetitive strain injuries, postural problems, muscle tension, osteoarthritis pain, sciatica, and sports concerns for runners and athletes like piriformis syndrome, tennis elbow, fibromyalgia, and upper-back or neck pain.

Contraindications for a Deep-Tissue Massage

What are the contraindications for a deep-tissue massage? The contraindications for a deep-tissue massage are the following:

- Atherosclerosis—a buildup of plaque in the artery walls
- Arteriosclerosis—hardening of the arteries
- Autoimmune diseases such as
  1. Lupus,
  2. Rheumatoid arthritis during inflammatory stage,

3. Scleroderma (hardened skin) during inflammatory stage, and

4. Ankylosing spondylitis—inflammation of tissues around the spine.

- Bipolar disorder
- Borderline
- Cerebral palsy
- Cancer (only if approved by a physician)
- Connective tissue disease
- Diabetes
- Embolism or thrombus
- Epileptics
- Headaches especially migraines
- Heart conditions
- Hemangioma
- Herpes and warts
- High blood pressure
- Impaired elimination system
- Intervertebral disc problems
- IUD (For deep abdominal work on female clients, IUD may get displaced!)
- Menstruation with very heavy bleeding
- Nose work, special conditions
- Pain medication
- Pregnancy
- Varicose veins
- Whiplash if inflamed

As a rule of thumb, never do deep work at all for conditions such as the following:

- Abscess teeth
- Aneurysm
- Bone fractures or acute soft tissue injuries
- Recent cortisone injection (wait two to three months)
- Fever

- Hemophiliacs
- Hodgkin's disease
- Inflammatory conditions such as tendonitis and bursitis
- Infectious conditions
- Leukemia
- Osteoporosis
- Phlebitis
- Recent scar tissue from surgeries, such as regular and plastic surgeries (wait until six weeks after surgery to receive a massage)

Shiatsu

Shiatsu is a massage technique that uses rhythmic pressure on precise points on the body called acupressure points, the massage therapist uses "finger pressure," which is the meaning of the Japanese word *shiatsu*. This type of massage helps unblock acu-points for a more enhanced flow of energy.

What Is Shiatsu Massage?

Shiatsu massage is when the massage therapist uses fingers, thumbs, and palms to apply pressure to certain areas of the body to help with certain ailments and conditions and to help correct any imbalances in the body. When pressure is applied to certain areas of the body, it helps promote energy flow and helps correct any disharmonies within the body. Shiatsu practitioners believe that when a person has a physical health condition or a disease, it is caused by blockages and an imbalance in the energy flow with in the body. However, once the energy becomes more balanced and there are no more blockages within the body, the body will then be able to heal itself.

History of Shiatsu Massage

So where did shiatsu massage originate from? Shiatsu massage originated from Japan by the founder Tokujiro Namikoshi, who at the age of seven years old, helped to care for his mother who was suffering from rheumatoid arthritis. While he was working with his mother, he used only his thumbs, fingers, and palms by applying pressure to certain areas of her body in 1912, which was the very beginning of shiatsu!

Later on in his life, he opened his own clinic in Sapporo in 1925 and opened another clinic in Tokyo in 1933. Then in 1940, he established his own school called The Japan Shiatsu College in Tokyo.

Benefits of Shiatsu Massage

What are the benefits of shiatsu massage? The benefits of shiatsu massage are the following: helps restore and maintain the body's energy; improves circulation; helps reduce stress, tension, anxiety, and depression; relieves headaches; promotes healing from sprains; relieves arthritis, stiffness in neck, shoulders, and back as well as sciatica, coughs, colds and sinus issues, insomnia, digestive issues, morning sickness, and menstrual problems.

Contraindications for Shiatsu Massage

What are the contraindications of shiatsu massage? The contraindications of shiatsu massage are the following:

- Fever
- Infectious skin diseases or open wounds
- Immediately after a surgery
- Cesarean birth (must be six months after the birth so abdomen can heal)
- Prone to blood clots
- Recent bruises, inflamed skin, unhealed wounds, abdominal hernia, or areas of recent fractures
- After a stroke or a cerebrovascular accident (wait six months after and consult a doctor especially if client/patient has suffered a stroke in the last two years)

- Diabetes (make sure client/patient gets regular checkups for sensory neuropathy)
- Certain medications (especially if client/patient is taking medication for thrombocytopenia and the medication is not working or only works intermittently)

Aromatherapy Massage

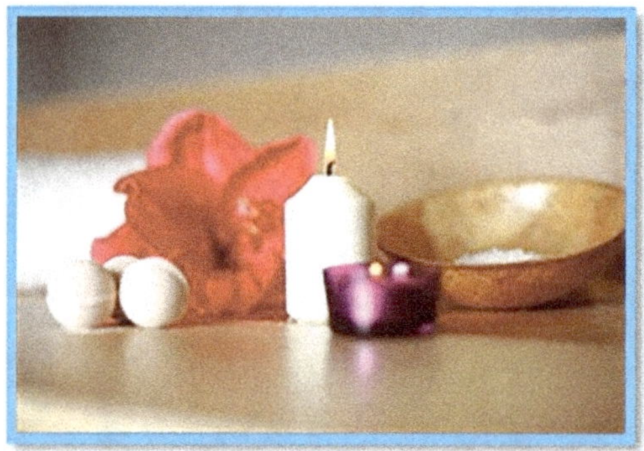

Aromatherapy is the use of essential oils. The scents of which stimulate the olfactory system, bringing various benefits including stress relief, relaxation, and a variety of other health benefits.

What Is Aromatherapy?

Aromatherapy is commonly used to help the body unwind, cure minor ailments, reduce stress levels, improve mood, and renew energy. There are a few ways to include aromatherapy into your life such as inhaling essential oils, adding them to your bath, and mixing them with a carrier oil to be used in massage therapy. For aromatherapy used in massage therapy, the pressure that is used is usually light to medium.

History of Aromatherapy

Where did aromatherapy originate from? Aromatherapy first originated from the Egyptians who developed one of the first distillation machines to extract oils from certain plants such as cedar wood, clove, and cinnamon. The oils were used to preserve or embalm the dead. They also used an herbal mixture called *kyphi*. Kyphi was a mixture of sixteen ingredients that could be used as incense, perfume, or medicine. Only the priests were allowed to use the aromatic oils, as they were believed to be one with the Gods.

In 2697–2597 BC, the use of aromatic oils was first recorded in China by Huang Ti. Huang Ti was the Yellow Emperor and he wrote a book called *The Yellow Emperor's Book of Internal Medicine*, which is still used today by practitioners who study Eastern medicine.

Later on, the uses of aromatherapy begin to spread to other places such as India, Greece, Rome, Persia, and Europe. In 1928 a French chemist Rene'-Maurice Gattefosse' wrote a book called, "Aromatherapie" based on his own experience with the aromatic oil Lavender.

One day, while he was working in his Laboratory, he had a small explosion and one of his hands got badly burned. He put his hand in liquid solution not realizing it was Lavender, and found out that Lavender was able to heal his hand without infections or scars.

What is aromatherapy used for? Aromatherapy is used for relaxation and stress relief. Plus, it can help with physical and mental conditions such as burns, infections, depression, insomnia, and high blood pressure.

Aromatherapy is also the use of essential oils from certain plants, herbs, roots, leaves, seeds, and blossoms that can be either inhaled or massaged into the skin. Essential oils should NEVER be taken by mouth unless you have specific instruction to do so from a qualified Specialist.

How does aromatherapy work? Researchers are not 100 percent sure how aromatherapy works, however there is a theory that the smell receptors in the nose communicates with parts of the brain such as the amygdala and hippocampus that serve both emotions and memories. So when you breathe in the essential oils, the oil stimulates the parts of your brain that influences physical, emotional, and mental health. For example, Lavender stimulates the brain cells that are very similar to the way some sedative medications would work, causing the person to feel very relaxed and sleepy.

Benefits of Aromatherapy

What are the benefits of aromatherapy? The benefits of aromatherapy are the following: helps relieve stress, can act as an antidepressant, boosts memory, increases energy levels, helps speed up healing, reduces headaches, regulates sleep, strengthens the immune system, relieves pain, and improves digestion.

The essential oils for stress are as follows:

- Lemon oil
- Lavender
- Bergamot
- Peppermint
- Vetiver
- Ylang-ylang

For antidepressant, the oils are as follows:

- Peppermint
- Chamomile
- Lavender
- Jasmine

For improving memory, the oil is as follows:

- Sage

For increasing energy, the oils are as follows:

- Black pepper

- Cardamom
- Cinnamon
- Clove
- Angelica
- Jasmine
- Tea Tree
- Rosemary
- Sage

For speeding up healing, the oils are as follows:

- Lavender
- Calendula
- Everlasting
- Buckthorn

For reducing headaches, the oils are as follows:

- Peppermint
- Eucalyptus
- Sandalwood
- Rosemary

For regulating sleep, the oils are as follows:

- Lavender
- Chamomile
- Jasmine
- Benzoin
- Neroli
- Sandalwood
- Sweet marjoram
- Ylang-ylang

For strengthening the immune system, the oils are as follows:

- Oregano
- Frankincense
- Lemon
- Peppermint
- Cinnamon
- Eucalyptus

For pain relief, the oils are as follows:

- Lavender
- Chamomile
- Clary Sage
- Juniper
- Eucalyptus
- Rosemary
- Peppermint

For improving digestion, the oils are as follows:

- Ginger
- Dill
- Fennel
- Chamomile
- Clary sage
- Lavender

A word of caution when using essential oils, it is always wise, when working with essential oils, that you use two to three drops with lotion or oil before applying to your skin. Why? A lot of the essential oils can be very strong and can irritate your skin!

Contraindications for Aromatherapy

What are the contraindications for aromatherapy? The contra-indications for aromatherapy are the following:

- Heart conditions
- Hypertension
- Cancer
- Epilepsy
- Allergic reactions
- Pregnancy
- Babies and children less than five years old
- Clients who are undergoing chemotherapy or who are feeling very ill such as severe nausea

Hot-Stone Massage

Hot-stone massage refers to a technique in which smooth, heated river stones are positioned on specific parts of the body in order to maximize the healing effect of the massage.

What Is Hot-Stone Massage?

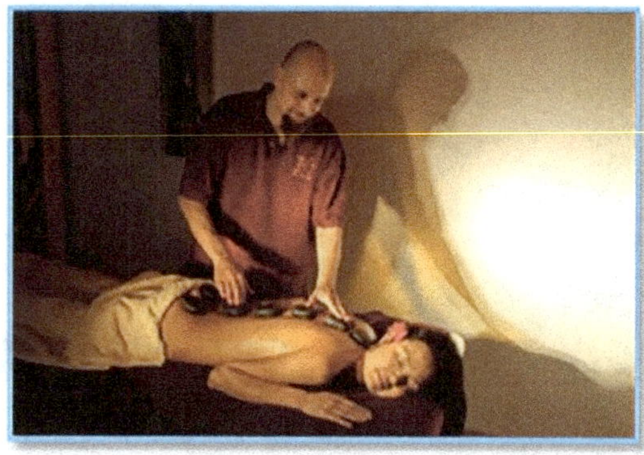

A hot-stone massage is when the massage therapist uses the heated stones as an extension of the massage therapist's hands—meaning that the massage therapist won't just leave the stones on the body but also that the massage therapist will actually glide and apply pressure with the stones. The pressure used for hot-stone massage is usually light to medium.

The purpose of these stones is to relax tense muscles, which is easily achieved through the weight and warmth of the stones.

History of Hot-Stone Massage

Where did hot-stone massage originate from? Hot-stone massage originated from the ancient Chinese medical practitioners as well as the Native Americans and the Hawaiians.

In 1993, hot-stone massage started gaining popularity and was introduced to the United States as being "rediscovered" by a massage therapist whose name was Mary Nelson. Mary Nelson was having a lot of pain in her shoulders and wrists due to repetitive injuries from giving massages. So one day she and her niece went to a sauna, and while she was in the sauna, she discovered the stones laying there and picked them up and started to massage herself with one as well as her niece. They both discovered that it felt great to the client as well as the massage therapist. Thus, hot-stone massage was discovered and the first style or name was called La Stone Therapy.

Benefits of a Hot-Stone Massage

What are the benefits of a hot-stone massage? The benefits of a hot-stone massage are that it is comforting, deeply relaxing, can be helpful to people who feel cold, have a lot of muscle tension, and who prefer a lighter touch. Also, hot-stone massage can help with other conditions such as the following:

- Anxiety
- Back pain
- Depression
- Insomnia
- Osteoarthritis

Contraindications for a Hot-Stone Massage

What are the contraindications for a hot-stone massage? The contraindications for a hot-stone massage are as follows:

- Blood clots/prone to blood clots

- Bruise easily
- Cancer, chemotherapy, or radiation treatments
- Depressed immune system (lupus, AIDS, HIV, cancer, Epstein-Barr virus, mononucleosis, etc…)
- Diabetes
- Fever
- Heart problems
- Heat sensitivity
- Inflamed skin conditions
- Nerve trauma
- Neuropathy
- Open wounds or sores
- Peripheral vascular disorder
- Pregnancy
- Recent surgery
- Taking medications that have side effects to heat
- Varicose veins

Reflexology

Most people believe that reflexology is just a fancy term for foot massage. However, reflexology is something much more. Reflexology has many health benefits that can help with cancer, arthritis, hypertension, type 2 diabetes, migraine, tension headaches, anxiety, depression, and sinusitis. It also helps eliminate toxins.

What Is Reflexology?

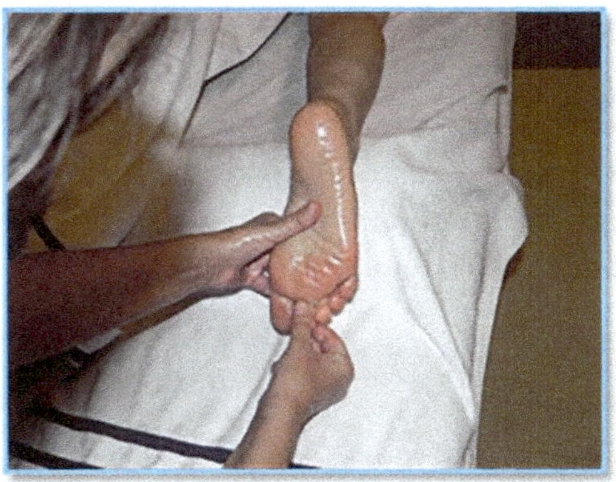

Reflexology is when the massage therapist applies pressure on specific reflex zones on the feet in order to induce a healing response in corresponding areas of the body. Usually, the pressure for reflexology is medium to firm.

History of Reflexology

Where did reflexology originate from? Reflexology originated from Egypt and China, and later it was introduced to America in the year 1913 by a doctor named William H. Fitzgerald who was an ear, nose, and throat specialist and by another man by the name of Edwin F. Bowers. Dr. Fitzgerald believed that applying pressure to an area on the body had an anesthetic effect on other parts of the body. This means that you temporarily felt no pain or sensation on other parts of the body.

Edwin Frederick Bowers was an American alternative medicine proponent, and together he and Dr. Fitzgerald invented "zone therapy." Zone therapy is when the body is divided by vertical lines into five zones on the left side of the body and five zones on the right side of the body. The idea is that energy runs up and down between all the parts of the body, and in order to have good health, the energy needs to be free-flowing and not blocked. If there is a blockage of energy, the organ will be affected—causing an imbalance of energy which could cause an illness.

What is reflexology? Reflexology is thought to be believed that there are certain pressure points on the ears, hands, and feet that correspond to other muscles and organs of the body. For example, the base of the little toe corresponds or represents the ear, and the ball of the foot corresponds or represents the lung.

Benefits of Reflexology

What are the benefits of reflexology? Reflexology can help relieve pain—such as neck pain, migraines, headaches, and upper- and lower-back pain—stimulate seven thousand nerve endings in the body, and fight anxiety and depression. For example, having the tops of your toes massaged can help enhance the production of serotonin in the adrenal, hypothalamic, pineal, and pituitary glands. Additionally, it helps improve circulation of blood throughout the body, improves foot health by reducing pain in the ankles and heels by keeping the ankles strong and flexible, promotes relaxation and better sleep, reduces PMS and menopausal symptoms for women, lowers blood pressure, provides relief from cancer-treatment side effects, and helps the body detox by improving the function of the bladder—making it more efficient in eliminating toxins and other waste products.

Contraindications for Reflexology

What are the contraindications for reflexology? The contraindications of reflexology are as follows:

- Foot fractures
- Unhealed wounds
- Active gout
- Osteoarthritis on foot or ankle
- Vascular disease of legs or feet
- Pregnancy (in the first six weeks)
- Thrombosis or embolism
- Open wounds

Sports Massage

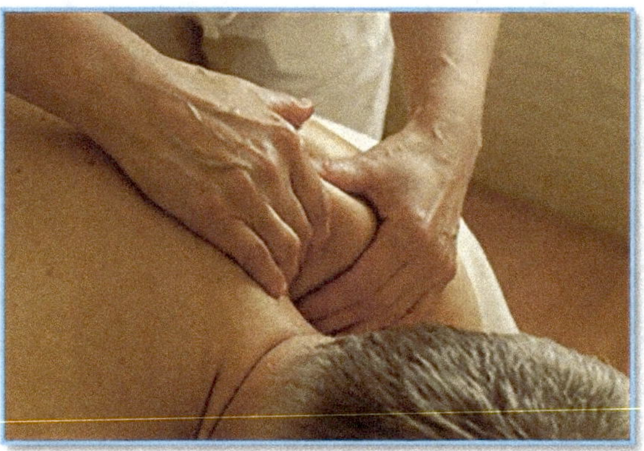

Sports massage is somewhat similar to deep-tissue massage therapy, simply because it also focuses on reaching the deeper layers of the muscle tissues.

What Is Sports Massage?

A sports massage is when a massage therapist uses different techniques to focus on specific areas of the body that are stressed and overworked from repetitive movements. The different techniques that are used during a sports massage are deep-tissue, trigger-point pressure, cross fiber, friction strokes, compression, and jostling.

Deep-tissue is when the massage therapist uses firm pressure and slow strokes to reach into the deeper layers of the muscles and the fascia.

Trigger-point pressure is when the massage therapist applies pressure to a certain area of pain in the body using elbows, feet, or other tools to apply direct pressure without overworking their hands.

Cross fiber is a technique that aims at breaking down knots and lesions in the muscles caused by injuries such as tears, breaks, and sprains.

Friction strokes is when the massage therapist works with their thumbs to break up adhesions deep into the muscle tissue and helps break apart and realign the muscle fibers.

Compression is when the massage therapist applies light to deep pressure on the muscles by laying their hands over a large muscle group and pushing down into the muscle tissues. For example, the massage therapist will lay their hands on a muscle group and then push down on the muscle tissue and then move to another muscle group and repeat the process so that the muscles are being held and released. The purpose of compressions is to help with relaxation, tight muscles, and acute pain relief.

Jostling is when the massage therapist lifts the muscle and gently shakes it in a rapid motion. It is very similar to rocking; however, rocking is much slower than jostling and is usually done in an up-or-down, side-to-side, and circular motions. The purpose of jostling is to help with muscle stiffness and muscle cramping especially in the calves for Athletes who train/practice in hot and humid weather conditions.

History of Sports Massage

Where did sports massage originate from? Sports massage originated from the ancient Greeks. The Greeks found that massage was very beneficial to the athletes before and after their Olympic games and to the warriors as well. The events that took place at the Olympics were wrestling, shot put, high jump, broad jump, and warring activities.

Later on in the 1960s, sports massage began to develop in the Soviet Union by the Russians for different Olympic games and international competitions. So then sports massage gained a lot of popularity throughout Europe and other countries as well. Then in the 1970s, sports massage gained popularity in the United States by an incredible performance at the 1972 Olympic Games by Finnish track-and-field athlete Lasse Virén who won both the 5,000- and 10,000-meter runs by receiving deep friction massages daily!

Who was the founder of sports massage? The founder of sports massage was Jack Meagher. Jack was a massage therapist who worked with humans and horses as well. He was a graduate of two massage therapy schools and a graduate of Physical Therapy. In 1985, he wrote a book called *Sports Massage* for massage therapists, students, and athletes. He also worked for the United States Equestrian Teams in Montreal for the Olympics in 1976 as well as other world championships in the United States and around the world. He was awarded the USET Certificate of Achievement and an honorary membership by the American Massage Therapy Association. Last but not the least, he conducted seminars about massages for both humans and horses throughout the United States and Canada and had publications of *Beating Muscle Injuries for Horses* and *Muscle Injuries for Runners*.

Benefits of Sports Massage

What are the benefits of sports massage? The benefits of sports massage are that it improves performance, reduces pain, prevents injuries, and helps shorten recovery time. Plus, it also promotes the growth of new mitochondria which is the energy-producing units in the cells. So not only does sports massage feel good but it is also good for the muscles.

Contraindications for Sports Massage

What are the contraindications for sports massage? The contra-indications for sports massage are the following:

- Fever
- Acute soft tissue inflammation
- High blood pressure

- Infectious diseases
- Hernia
- Osteoporosis
- Varicose veins
- Fractures
- Skin diseases
- Deep vein thrombosis (DVT)
- Recent surgery
- Myositis ossificans
- Pregnancy

Lymph Massage

Also referred to as lymphatic drainage, lymph massage was designed to help eliminate your body's waste. Lymphatic massage is typically the treatment of choice for swollen tissues as it helps remove proteins and waste products from the affected area and reduce the swelling.

What Is Lymph Massage?

Lymph massage is a massage that uses very light pressure with long, gentle, rhythmic strokes and with soft pumping movements in the direction of the lymph nodes. Usually, the massage therapist will start at the feet and work up the rest of the body.

History of Lymph Massage

Where did lymph massage originate from? Lymph massage originated from France by two founders, Emil Vodder, PhD, and his wife, Estrid Vodder. Emil Vodder was born in the year 1896 in Copenhagen, Denmark. Later, he went onto the University of Copenhagen and took courses and/or classes in biology, mineralogy, botany, medicine, cytology, and microscopy. Plus, he also had an interest in learning physical medicine.

Then, near the end of the eighth semester, he had contacted malaria and was not permitted to finishing his studies in medicine. However, in 1928, he did earn a PhD at the University of Brussels for his thesis on historical art.

So in 1933, Vodder and his wife, Estrid, moved to Paris, France, and studied anatomy and physiology of the lymph vessel system within the body. They also worked with patients who had chronic sinusitis, chronic colds, and other immune disorders. They discovered that these patients all had swollen lymph nodes. So they developed a massage technique that involved a light, rhythmic hand movement to help with lymph movement or flow within the body.

In 1936, Vodder called his technique a Manual Lymph Drainage during a congress in Paris, France. Later in the 1950s, Vodder started to receive a lot of invitations from other European countries to teach his Manual Lymph Drainage technique. Then in 1966, Gunther Wittlinger came in contact with Dr. Vodder and founded the first Dr. Vodder School in 1972 in Walchsee, Austria.

In New York, in 1972, the Dr. Vodder technique was introduced in North America by Hildegard and Gunther Wittlinger at a conference. Ten years later, they went back to Toronto, Canada and began to train therapists and met with Robert Harris, which was the director of the Dr. Vodder School-International. The Dr. Vodder School was founded in 1993, in North America and today is taught in other countries such as Australia, Singapore, Japan, New Zealand, Ireland, UK, and other European countries.

Benefits of Lymph Massage

What are the benefits of lymph massage? The benefits of lymph massage are it can help reduce the chances of getting minor colds and viruses, help the body to fight off infections, speed up healing and recovery from an illness, reduce water retention, and boost weight loss. Also, it can improve skin texture by reducing puffiness and blotches, cleaning out pores, speeding up healing in scar tissue, and reducing cellulite.

Lymphatic massage is especially relaxing and pleasant because it helps reduce pain all over the body. According to the International Alliance of Healthcare Educators, this particular massage therapy promotes general wellness, vitality, and healing.

Healing after Surgery

Lymph drainage massage is supportive of healing following surgery as it regenerates tissues to reduce scarring that occurs as a result of surgical incisions. This therapy also reduces swelling, regenerates tissues and cells, and helps detox the body, as reported by the International Alliance of Healthcare Educators. Lymph massage should take place no sooner than six weeks following surgery and after a doctor has given approval.

Improved Breastfeeding

Breastfeeding complications as result of improper latching may include sore nipples, engorged breasts, and pain. Lymphatic massage can help reduce the swelling that results from engorgement and help ameliorate plugged ducts, resulting in less pain of the nipples and breasts and leading to better breastfeeding.

Improved Immune System Functioning

Lymph massage helps improve immune function and stimulates the production of antibodies that help fight off infection and disease, and it goes further to reduce inflammation inside the body that is linked to various chronic conditions, such as arthritis.

Contraindications for Lymph Massage

What are the contraindications for lymph massage? The contraindications of a lymph massage are the following:

- Congestive heart failure
- Acute renal failure
- Active blood clots
- Active infection
- Active bleeding
- Undiagnosed cancer

Healing Touch/Energy-Healing Massage

Healing touch is an energy therapy that revolves around the use of gentle hand techniques in order to help re-pattern the energy field of the patient, thus helping him or her accelerate healing of the mind, body, and spirit.

The two types of energy work are therapeutic touch and Reiki. These are all based on a theory that people are fields of energy that constantly interact with other people and the environment.

What Is Therapeutic Touch?

Therapeutic Touch is a form of energy work where the practitioner starts at the head of the client and moves down the body towards the toes, hovering their hands over the body—about two to four inches above the body by not touching it. It is from an ancient practice called laying on of hands. The purpose of therapeutic touch is to help correct or balance the energy fields within the body. So if a person is in good health, it means that the energy within the body is balanced. Whereas, if a person has an illness, it means that the energy within the body is unbalanced. The energy fields in the body are considered to be life energy; the life energy in the body helps maintain normal functions such as physiological, psychological, and spiritual. In Chinese medicine, this energy field is called qi, which is pronounced "chee." In Ayurveda medicine, the energy field is called prana.

History of Therapeutic Touch

Where did therapeutic touch originate from? Therapeutic touch originated from the Egyptians, Chinese, Indians, Polynesians, Native Americans, Greeks, Romans, and Africans. Therapeutic touch was used for early Shaman practices, traditional healing practices, and the practices of religions including Christianity.

The founders of therapeutic touch were two women by the names of Dolores Krieger PhD, RN and Dora Kunz. Dolores Krieger PhD, RN was a professor of Nursing and Dora Kunz was a natural healer. They both discovered therapeutic touch in the early 1970s. They first taught the techniques to the graduates at the New York University of Nursing. Later it began to gain popularity among other nurses due to Krieger's research and writings about it.

Benefits of Therapeutic Touch

What are the benefits for therapeutic touch? The benefits of therapeutic touch are it helps relieve stress, boosts the immune system, relieves pain, heals wounds, and increases oxygen in red blood cells to help carry out oxygen throughout the body. It can also be very beneficial to those who have had amputations done to their extremities. Research has shown that people who have had their leg, arm, hand, or foot amputated can still feel sensations. A lot of these sensations are known as phantom pain. So as a massage therapist, if you come across someone who has had an amputation of their extremity, it would be best to massage that area as if it is still there. Why? The person who has had an amputation done can actually "feel" what you are doing. Plus if the "phantom pain" is severe, it can help ease that pain and promote relaxation.

Contraindications for Therapeutic Touch

What are the contraindications for therapeutic touch? There are no contraindications for therapeutic touch. However, it is advisable for the practitioner to use caution with clients who have fever or acute inflammation going on in their body and clients who have a history of physical or sexual Abuse. Also, it is advisable when working with clients who are children, elderly, and debilitated to make the session brief.

Reiki

Reiki is a Japanese technique for stress reduction and relaxation that also promotes healing.

What Is Reiki?

Reiki is very similar to therapeutic touch. However, the practitioner actually touches the client with their hands. This technique is called palm healing or hands-on healing, which is transferred from the practitioner to the client with universal energy.

History of Reiki

Where did Reiki originate from? Reiki originated from Japan in 1922 by a Japanese Buddhist by the name of Mikao Usui. Mikao Usui was born in 1865 and died in 1926. One day while he was teaching in a College, a student came to him and asked him how Jesus was able to perform miracles. Moved by that question, he went out on a quest to find the answer to that question. He traveled to the holy mountains of Kori Yama to attain a high-altered state of consciousness by meditating and fasting for twenty-one days. Then on the twenty-first day, as he was about to give up on his quest, he was enlightened by a great spiritual energy on the top of his head. This energy was Reiki Ryoho, which is a healing energy.

Mikao Usui felt that Reiki was a Spiritual practice and felt that it was an opportunity for people to awaken their true natures. Even though Mikao Usui was the original founder of Reiki, two other people followed his footsteps. They were Dr. Chujiro Hayashi and Mrs. Hawayo Takata.

Dr. Chujiro Hayashi was one of Mikao Usui's students who opened a clinic in 1940. He studied with Mikao for ten months before he died. He also was a retired naval officer and a surgeon.

Mrs. Hawayo Takata was a Japanese descent who was born in Hawaii in 1900. She lost both her husband and sister and began to have poor health. Since she was having poor health, she decided to go to Japan to find a doctor that would help her. She found a doctor in Japan who felt that she needed surgery. She felt strongly against that, so the doctor referred her to Dr. Hayashi's clinic.

After receiving weekly treatments at the clinic, her health began to improve and she was really amazed by Dr. Hayashi's work and wanted to learn more about it. So he taught her Reiki I and Reiki II and studied with her from 1936–1938.

When she came back to Hawaii from Japan, she practiced Reiki and opened her own clinic. In the 1970s she began to train Reiki masters, and in 1980, the year of her death, she had trained a total of twenty-two Reiki masters!

Benefits of Reiki

What are the benefits of Reiki? The benefits of Reiki are it reduces stress, creates relaxation, helps bring feelings of inner peace and harmony, balances the mind and emotions, offers relief from distress (emotional) and sorrow such as grief, and relieves pain from migraine, headaches, arthritis, and sciatica. It also helps with asthma, chronic fatigue, menopausal symptoms (for women), insomnia, speeds up recovery from surgery or an illness, reduces side effects from treatments such as chemotherapy, and helps with problems that are both physical and mental. Plus, Reiki can be used on adults, babies, toddlers, children, elderly, and pets.

Contraindications for Reiki

What are the contraindications for Reiki? The contraindications for Reiki are the following:

- During a surgery. It is best to receive Reiki before or after surgery.
- Broken bones. It is best to wait until a doctor puts a cast on the broken bone or bones first. Then the person can receive Reiki treatments for healing.
- Amputations. It is best to wait for a medical procedure or surgery of the body part before doing Reiki on a client. Otherwise, the wound could close too quickly, making it impossible for the doctor to do the procedure.

Pregnancy Massage

Pregnancy massage is a massage that helps improve circulation and helps you relax. It can reduce anxiety, relieve muscle aches, improve sleep, and increase the feel-good hormones such as serotonin and dopamine—which can improve the pregnant woman's mood by giving her a sense of well-being.

What Is Pregnancy Massage?

Pregnancy massage is a massage that helps improve circulation and promotes relaxation. The pressure performed during a pregnancy massage is usually light to medium.

History of Pregnancy Massage

Where did pregnancy massage originate from? Pregnancy massage originated from India and Africa.

Who was the founder of pregnancy massage? The founder of pregnancy massage was a woman by the name of Carole Osborne-Sheets. Carole Osborne-Sheets researched the developing infant and prenatal massage with perinatal professionals and colleagues. One of the perinatal professionals and colleagues was a man by the name of Dr. George Engelmann. Dr. George Engelmann was a professor of obstetrics in postgraduate school of Missouri Pathological Societies and consulting surgeon at St. Louis Female Hospital. Dr. George Engelmann wrote a lot of articles in medical journals about the positive effects of receiving prenatal massages.

So in 1980, Carole started to develop infant and pregnancy massage therapy protocols and instructional programs and/or classes. Ever since then, she has trained parents, hospital staff, and four thousand prenatal massage therapists!

Benefits of Pregnancy Massage

What are the benefits for pregnancy massage? The benefits of pregnancy massage are it can reduce anxiety, decrease the symptoms of depression, help relieve muscle aches and joint pain, help improve labor as well as promote healthy newborns, reduce swelling, improve nerve pain such as sciatica, reduce headaches, and improve sleep.

Contraindications for Pregnancy Massage

What are the contraindications of pregnancy massage? The contraindications for a pregnancy massage are as follows:

- High-risk pregnancies
- Pregnancy-induced hypertension (PIH)
- Preeclampsia
- Previous preterm labor
- Severe swelling
- High blood pressure
- Severe headache
- Recently gave birth (before six weeks)

Geriatric Massage

Geriatric massage is a massage that is given to the elderly using gentle and light pressure. This is very similar to a Swedish massage.

What Is Geriatric Massage?

Geriatric massage is the use of gentle hand motions, passive movements, and gentle stretching. For example, stretching of the shoulders, legs, and feet helps improve joint mobility and flexibility. It is also the gentle massaging of the hands and feet and sometimes the use of friction and pressure strokes near the shoulders.

History of Geriatric Massage

Where did geriatric massage originate from? Geriatric massage originated from Sweden in the 1850s.

Who was the founder of geriatric massage? There were actually two founders, and they were two brothers by the names of Dr. Charles and Dr. George Taylor.

What Are the Benefits of Geriatric Massage?

The benefits of geriatric massage are it helps increase blood circulation, improves the lymphatic flow to help the body get rid of toxins, helps with headaches and pain, speeds up healing from an injury or an illness, improves quality of sleep, relieves stress, anxiety, depression, and loneliness, and helps improve self-esteem and quality of life.

What Are the Contraindications for Geriatric Massage?

The contraindications for a geriatric massage are the following:

- Broken bones, inflammation, swelling, bruises
- Bed sores—either open or not healed
- Recent surgery
- Acute or severe pain
- Heart conditions
- Cancer
- Blood clots
- Blood thinner drugs

The Benefits of Massage

Massage benefits the body, mind, and spirit in many ways.

General Health

The general health benefits of massage are the following:

- Promotes delivery of nutrients and oxygen cells within the muscle
- Helps remove waste products
- Circulatory effects help in treating inflammatory conditions, such as arthritis or edema through the use of lymphatic massage
- Induces the relaxation response to lower heart rate and reduced blood pressure and respiration rate and alleviate the many side effects of stress to promote a calm and healing environment within the body. Stress reduction and well-managed stress can also prevent the many chronic conditions associated with it, such as heart disease, depression, and anxiety.
- Relaxes and calms the mind and spirit to make you more productive and generally better equipped to handle life

Mobility and Movement

Massage relaxes muscle tissue to decrease nerve compression, increase joint space, and improve range of motion, leading to improved functioning and easier movement.

Enhanced Blood Flow and Blood Circulation

Enhanced blood flow and blood circulation is one of the notable health benefits of many types of massage techniques such as Swedish and deep-tissue, which use strokes that move toward and away from the heart, thereby increasing blood circulation throughout the body. For example, if you were suffering from poor circulation, you would have discomforts like fatigue, cold hands, cold feet, pooling of fluid in your extremities, and an accumulation of lactic acid in your muscles.

However, if you receive massages on a regular basis such as every two weeks to monthly, your blood circulation will improve and this, over time, will have an incredibly positive effect on your overall health—helping you feel relaxed and having lower blood pressure as well, if your blood pressure was high to begin with.

Medical Conditions Helped by Massage

Migraines and Headaches

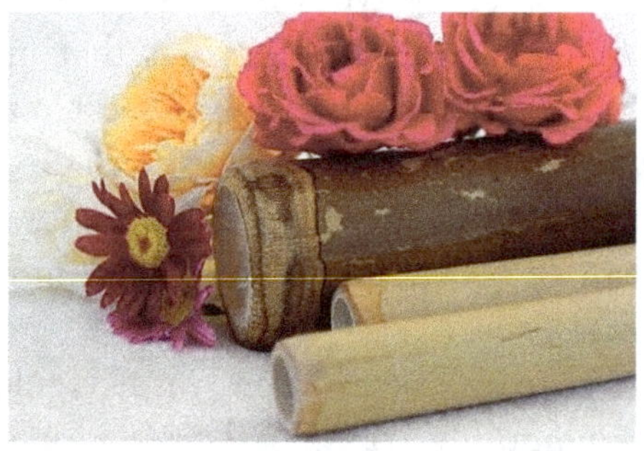

Many people suffer from migraines and chronic headaches. A lot of these headaches are caused by pain in the neck and shoulders, usually caused by physical or emotional stress, tension, anxiety, depression, and excitement. Suffering from these conditions can be quite exhausting, since it often leads to lack of sleep and higher stress levels. This is why many people turn to massage therapy to experience relief from headaches.

Diabetes

Diabetes is a disease marked by damage to insulin production of the pancreas and features various symptoms including excessive thirst, eye, heart, kidney, and nerve damage, frequent urination, and thickening of fascia that surrounds organs and muscles.

Massage can help those with both type 1 and type 2 diabetes in numerous ways. First, it promotes relaxation, which improves all of the body's internal functions. Second, massage improves circulation, which helps promote more efficient uptake of insulin. Massage also improves mobility and joint motion and decreases stiffness.

Parkinson's Disease

When an individual is suffering from Parkinson's disease, their central nervous system slowly begins to deteriorate. When your nerve cells die, your movement becomes affected. People who are suffering from Parkinson's disease often experience shaking and tremors as well as uncoordinated movement.

There are some medications that can help reduce these symptoms, but it's better if you throw massage therapy into the mix. Massage therapy can help reduce muscle spasms, which are present in people with Parkinson's. It can also improve the state of your nervous system and help you get more quality sleep.

Heart Health

Excessive stress can cause numerous health problems, including cardiac arrhythmias. Additionally, high blood pressure will increase the risk of a heart attack.

Thankfully, massage therapy is known for both stabilizing your blood pressure and reducing stress. According to the American Massage Therapy Association, massage significantly decreases heart rate, systolic blood pressure, and diastolic blood pressure. These are the major reasons that getting massages regularly can significantly improve your heart health.

Healthy Blood Pressure

The scary thing about high blood pressure is that it has absolutely no symptoms, which is why it's often referred to as the silent killer. This is exactly why you need to make sure you check your blood pressure often, especially as you get older.

There are a few ways to stave off high blood pressure, such as exercising, eating healthy, and getting massages regularly. Massage therapy is known for lowering blood pressure, which will in turn decrease your risk of suffering from a stroke, kidney failure, or a heart attack.

Fatigue

Every person experiences fatigue from time to time. Although fatigue isn't a cause for too much concern, as it usually goes away after you rest up, it can be a symptom of chronic fatigue syndrome, and it can certainly significantly lower your quality life.

Individuals who suffer from this syndrome can experience extreme fatigue for extended time periods, which can greatly affect their lifestyle. Massage therapy is currently one of the best alternative treatments for the symptoms of fatigue and chronic fatigue syndrome.

PTSD

Soldiers aren't the only people who can suffer from post-traumatic stress disorder. In fact, anyone who has ever experienced a severe trauma, such as abuse, crime, grief, or loss, can suffer from PTSD. The usual symptoms of this disorder include a feeling of detachment, chronic pain, anger, insomnia, severe anxiety, nightmares, and flashbacks.

You experience these symptoms due to imbalances in certain brain chemicals caused by stress that results from extreme trauma.

Thankfully, engaging in massage therapy regularly is an efficient way to restore balance to these brain chemicals and to help reduce PTSD symptoms.

Asthma and Bronchitis

Even if you're not suffering from asthma, you probably have a hard time taking a deep breath when faced with a stressful situation. However, just imagine what it's like for people suffering from asthma. Considering that massage therapy is known for relaxing the respiratory muscles used in breathing, your life can change for the better if you start getting massages regularly.

Aromatherapy massages are especially helpful for people suffering from asthma, with the help of certain essential oils that help improve respiration and promote healthier breathing.

The eight essential oils for asthma are as follows:

- Peppermint
- Lavender
- Tea tree
- Eucalyptus
- Frankincense
- Oregano
- Clove
- Thyme

The seven essential oils for bronchitis are as follows:

- Tea tree
- Cinnamon bark
- Lemon grass
- Thyme essential oil
- Eucalyptus
- Rosemary oil
- Lavender
- Clove

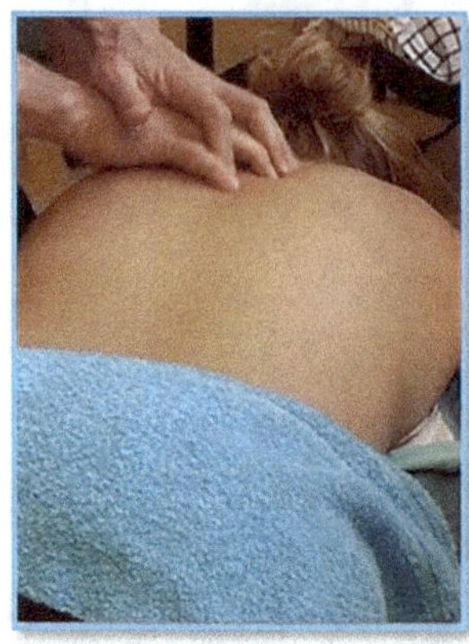

A note of caution, if you as a client is on antibiotics for bronchitis, check with your Doctor or a holistic doctor *first*. Some oils work well with antibiotics, and some do not. The risk with combining oils with antibiotics is that the antibiotics will become less effective, possibly making your condition worse!

Cancer and Cancer Treatment

Oncology massage is a modified form of massage whose purpose is to safely address complications of cancer and side effects of cancer treatment and to support the patient in anyway needed.

An oncology massage therapist receives specialized training in understanding the disease itself and the many ways it can affect the body, along with the side effects of various types of cancer treatment, such as chemotherapy, radiation, surgery, and medication.

A skilled therapist will modify massage techniques to meet the individual needs of the patient, in adaptation of their side effects and the various ways they are affected by the disease.

Insomnia

Due to chronic pain or high stress levels, it can be nearly impossible to get a good night's sleep. Watching the clock tick at night while you're wide awake can be extremely frustrating.

Starting off the day when you know that you haven't gotten enough sleep can also raise your stress levels, thus making your insomnia even more intense.

Insomnia is linked with increased risk of anxiety, depression, and memory loss. It is also one of the main causes of industrial disasters, medical errors, and car crashes.

Even though there are pills that will help you sleep, taking prescription medication can be addictive. Instead of taking sleeping pills to fix your insomnia problem, try getting regular massages.

Massages by a trained therapist can help alter the balance of neurochemicals in the brain, increasing expression of GABA (a key neurotransmitter for promoting restfulness) along with endorphins, which are key brain chemicals to combat the effect of adrenalin on the body, seeking to calm down neurons as the day progresses.

By informing your therapist about your insomnia issues, you will receive a massage tailored to help you deal with this condition.

Massage therapy is a great way to become more relaxed, reduce your stress levels, and relieve pain. All of this will help make your insomnia go away.

One way to address insomnia more effectively is to hire a therapist that will come to your home close to your bedtime as possible, to really relax you and prepare the body for a good night's sleep.

Recovery from Surgery

Surgery to fix a specific health problem is very important, but so is the recovery process. Proper post-surgery rehabilitation is essential if you want to start feeling as you did when you were healthy.

Massage therapy is an excellent way to make sure nutrients and blood reach the area of your body affected by the surgery and help in repairing the soft tissue.

Additionally, by getting massages, you will ensure that less scar tissue develops on your skin, such as the case with lymphatic massage. By improving circulation, the rehabilitating areas of your body will heal at a faster pace.

Immunity Health

Having a strong immune system will help keep you safe from a number of different diseases. Most people have an incredibly weak immune system, mostly due to the lifestyle they lead. If you're always dealing with a lot of stress and not eating properly, then your immune system will gradually start losing its ability to protect your body from harmful microorganisms.

Massage therapy is known for increasing the presence of your body's natural white blood cells, which will help you fight against infection and bacteria.

Dr. Gail Ironson, of the University of Miami, completed a study with a group of HIV-positive men being given a forty-five-minute massage, five days a week over the course of a month. These men saw a serotonin increase and an increase in the white blood cells that are viewed as our immune system's first line of defense.

As it heightens the immune systems response, massage is a natural painkiller. Studies have shown that just one massage will have an immediate benefit on your immune system, while regular massages offer a cumulative long-term benefit.

Massage lowers stress hormone levels while increasing white blood cell counts. It's a highly effective therapy for boosting immunity. It is one of the most enjoyable and affordable methods of staying healthy.

Improved Athletic Performance and Recovery

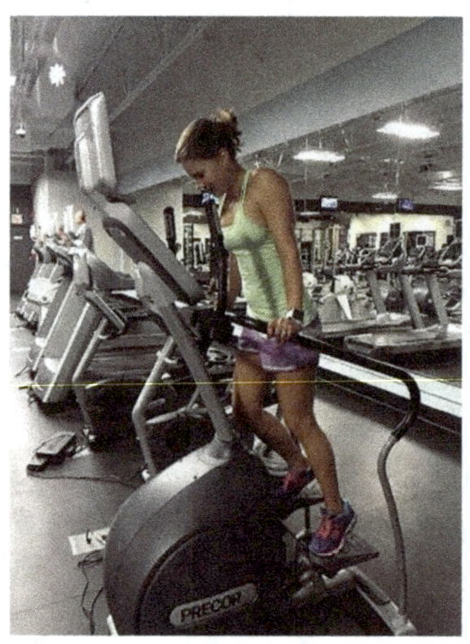

If you're a professional or an amateur athlete, massage therapy can help improve your athletic performance. There are several ways massage therapy can help with your athletic performance. For example, it can help with promoting flexibility, increasing range of motion, reducing fatigue, improving endurance, preventing injuries, and improving concentration or mental clarity.

The types of massages athletes use are sports massage and deep-tissue. Sports massage is a fast-paced massage used to help to stimulate the muscles. It can be used before a workout (pre-workout) and after a workout (post-workout). The techniques that are used are usually fast and the therapist may incorporate stretching as well. The benefits of sports massage are that it can get the muscles warmed up and stretched out and help get rid of any spasms. Deep-tissue massage is when the therapist works on specific problem areas by applying slow and heavy pressure on the muscle layers. This type of massage is designed to work out any knots and tension in the muscles.

Note that as a client, if you are about to do a long run (a marathon) or a tough workout, it is advisable to get a massage three to five days before the event and three to five days after the event to allow your muscles to recover.

Mental and Emotional Health Benefits

The Touch Research Institute of the University of Miami has led many studies on the benefits of massage for mental health, and results show it to be beneficial for various conditions, including the following:

- Anorexia nervosa
- Depression
- Stress
- Anxiety
- Various other mental health conditions

Improved Mood

Anyone who has ever had a professional massage knows that there is a huge difference in how you feel before and after visiting a massage therapist. There are numerous reasons as to why massage is known for improving your mood, such as reduced stress and increased levels of feel good chemicals, including serotonin and endorphins. Not to mention that you will feel much happier when you reach a state of deep relaxation.

Anxiety

According to the American Massage Therapy Association, massage therapy is known for assisting in the reduction of anxiety symptoms. Anxiety is basically caused by our body's natural response to danger, known as the fight-or-flight instinct.

However, this response to danger requires increased cortisol levels in order to make sure that your muscles are ready for the danger you're facing. Cortisol is also known as the stress hormone, and high levels of it can lead to a number of health problems.

A massage therapist can target areas of your body where you carry anxiety symptoms, thus lowering your cortisol levels.

Massage therapy will also improve your serotonin levels, which is a hormone that is known for elevating your mood.

According to the American Massage Therapy Association,

- massage reduces trait anxiety and depression providing benefits similar to those in magnitude as psychotherapy,
- massage increases neurotransmitters that are associated with lowering anxiety and decreases hormones that play a key role in increasing anxiety,
- massage lowers anxiety in cancer patients, and
- massage lowers anxiety and depression in military veterans.

Relaxation

According to AMTA 2015 consumer survey, 33 percent of responders reported getting a massage for stress reduction and relaxation.

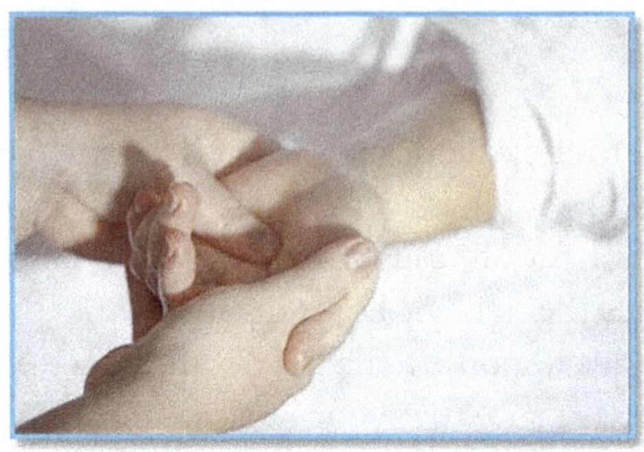

It's no secret that massage therapy can help you relax. In fact, that's one of the main reasons why most people even choose to get a massage. When the muscles in your body are tense, you can experience digestive problems, sleeplessness, and headaches.

All massage therapy techniques were designed specifically to help relax your tense muscles, thus making you reach a state of deep relaxation. Achieving this state will provide you with improved emotional health as well as better focus and memory.

Lower Stress Levels

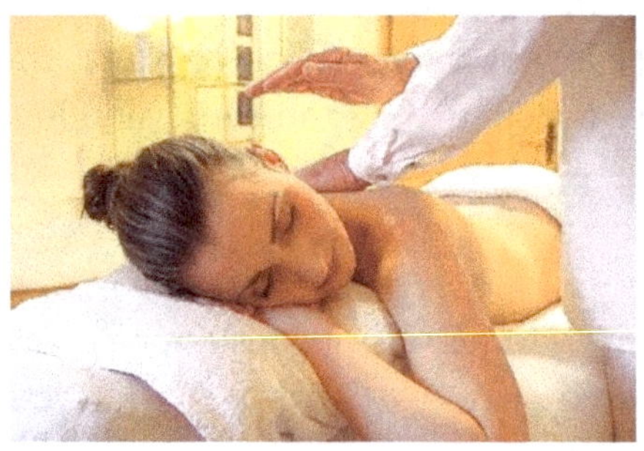

According to AMTA, massage is the most widely used type of complementary and alternative medicine in hospitals today for stress reduction and general well-being.

Stress is not always a bad thing. For example, if you're feeling energetic before an important meeting, then you're dealing with the good kind of stress. However, if you're constantly experiencing stress and when it becomes a chronic state, then that's when you should start to worrying.

When you experience continuous or chronic stress, your body is constantly flooded with stress hormones and remains in a constant state of distress known as fight-or-flight, which can lead to numerous health problems, including higher blood pressure, insomnia, headaches, heart disease, chest pain, depression, anxiety, body aches and reduced quality of life. It's also worth mentioning that stress is known for worsening the symptoms of certain diseases.

By taking part in massage therapy, and especially on a regular basis, you will reduce your stress levels, which will in turn lower your risk of suffering from numerous health conditions. Massage also stimulates the productions of endorphins, also known as feel-good chemicals. Lowering your stress levels will not only improve your physical health but it will also benefit your emotional health.

Researchers from the University of Miami School of medicine found that levels of the stress hormone cortisol were lowered by as much as 53 percent following just one session of massage.

According to Sandy Fritz, MS, NCTMB, author of a textbook line for therapeutic massage and director of the Health Enrichment Center in Lapeer, Michigan, "Research has shown that massage interfaces with the body's stress function" and "It helps to [*sic*] dampen the flight-or-fight response and activates dominance in the rest-and-restore system."

Depression

Massage therapy makes a great all-natural addition to depression management. The American Massage Therapy Association acknowledges that massage therapy is able to reduce the symptoms of this condition.

The reason why massage therapy can reduce the risk of depression is that it lowers your cortisol levels by as much as 50 percent.

Additionally, it raises levels of dopamine and serotonin, two neurotransmitters known for improving mood, and serotonin deficiency is a cause of major depression disorder.

According to the American Massage Therapy Association, massage also reduces depression in those who suffer from HIV.

Reduction in Anger and Aggression

You should never let stress lead you to your breaking point, as that can lead to depression, anxiety, anger, and aggression. However, you can avoid all of this simply by getting a massage once in a while. If you visit a massage therapist often, there probably won't be any chance for your stress levels to increase drastically.

Pain Conditions Helped by Massage

According to the AMTA 2015 consumer survey, 91 percent of people surveyed agree that massage can be effective in reducing pain.

Muscle Tension

Although some people experience muscle tension in the neck, back, and shoulders from exercising too much, most experience it due to excessive sitting. Improper posture while standing and sitting is one of the main causes of chronic back pain.

Thankfully, massage therapy is able to help you by relaxing your tense muscles and improving your flexibility.

Chronic Back Pain

A 2011 study that was published in the *Annals of Internal Medicine* reported evidence that massage is very effective for those who suffer from chronic back pain.

Chronic back pain is actually one of the most common reasons people get a massage, no matter its cause—be it poor posture, work-related and other injuries, stress, or carrying heavy items.

Fibromyalgia

Fibromyalgia is a very painful condition that affects the nerves of the body and makes life quite difficult for those suffering from it. Various massage therapies can help.

- Trigger point therapy targets the most painful spots, which are located in bands of muscle fibers. This type of massage deactivates these areas by targeting trigger points identified to be the source of most pain and uses pressure applied with the fingertip to massage them.
- Swedish massage helps fibromyalgia patients alleviate stress. This in turn helps promote relaxation and general well-being that helps with pain management.
- Myofascial release is a form of massage that applies gentle pressure to connective tissue and helps ease fibromyalgia pain by restoring motion by elongating muscle fibers.
- Hot-stone massage promotes relaxation and stress relief, thereby helping fibromyalgia sufferers reduce pain, improve their well-being and quality of life.
- Passive stretching is a practice where external force is placed on a limb in order to move it into a new position. Those who suffer from fibromyalgia will have very stiff joints, which are caused by constant muscle spasms featured in this condition. Passive stretching helps gently move extremities in the same direction to loosen tight joints and muscles.
- Sports massage can also benefit those with fibromyalgia as it releases stress and tension that builds up in the soft tissues of the body during physical activity. Sports massage also boosts blood circulation, reduces heart rate and blood pressure, increases lymph flow, improves flexibility, and eases pain.

It's a good idea to find a massage therapist experienced in dealing with fibromyalgia patients. One example are the clinical massage therapists who work in a medical facility or hospital, as these are experts in various medical conditions, including fibromyalgia and how it affects the body, so they will be able to create a sound and effective treatment plan.

Arthritis and Rheumatoid Arthritis

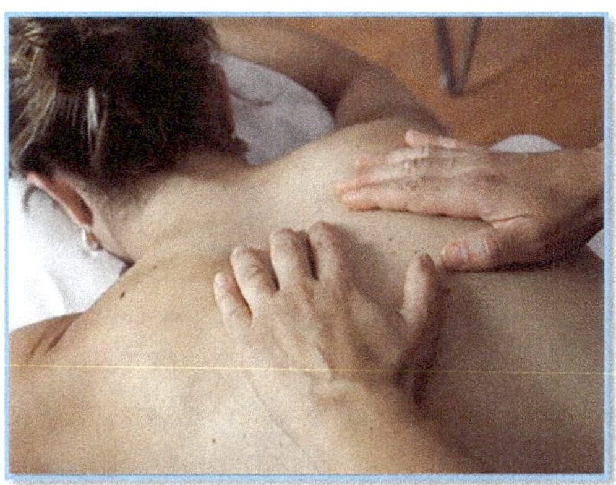

Suffering from arthritis can limit your normal activities.

Thankfully, massage therapy is known for reducing pain associated with this condition, as well as increase mobility for people suffering from arthritis.

Regular massages could improve grip strength, relieve pain, and reduce anxiety in people suffering from this condition.

Various massage therapies can help with arthritis; you can discuss options that are most fitting for your condition with your therapist:

- Swedish
- Deep-tissue
- Hot-stone
- Reflexology
- Shiatsu

Frozen Shoulder

If you're having difficulty lifting your arms high, then you may be suffering from a frozen shoulder or adhesive capsulitis. This condition is marked by soreness and stiffness within the shoulder joint and is considered to be very painful and debilitating. Frozen shoulder affects 5 percent of the population.

Basically, having a frozen shoulder means that the connective tissue around your shoulders tendons, ligaments, and bones became tighter.

Regular massage therapy and other bodywork modalities help treat this condition and alleviate the pain caused by it. Not only will it help with pain relief, but regular massages will also improve range of motion.

According to one study, deep friction massage can help frozen shoulder. Therapeutic massage techniques including trigger-point therapy, stretching and joint mobilization, and myofascial release either applied individually or in combination have shown positive results in alleviating frozen shoulder symptoms.

Massage techniques strive to release stiffness, boost blood and oxygen circulation, release locked-up muscles, and improve movement. A qualified massage therapist can create a treatment plan that consists of multiple sessions designed to unlock the stiff shoulder and restore the body's normal range of motion.

Sciatica

If you start experiencing pain from your lower back all the way down through your leg, then you may have damaged your sciatic nerve. This is one of the longer nerves found in the body, which is why the pain is so noticeable.

In sciatica, the tightening of the piriformis muscles in the back places undue stress on the nerve roots and massage helps loosen those muscles and also prevents irritation and pinching.

Furthermore, massage helps stimulate the release of the body's natural painkillers, known as endorphins to provide relief for sciatica symptoms, including throbbing pain in the foot and burning sensations in the legs.

Jeff Smoot, vice president of the American Massage Therapy Association says that trigger-point therapy is the best type of massage for sciatica. Trigger-point therapy applies pressure to the irritated and inflamed areas in the piriformis muscle, glutes, and lower back. Typically, progress can be seen by the fourth session, with treatments being given seven to ten days apart.

Rotator Cuff Syndrome

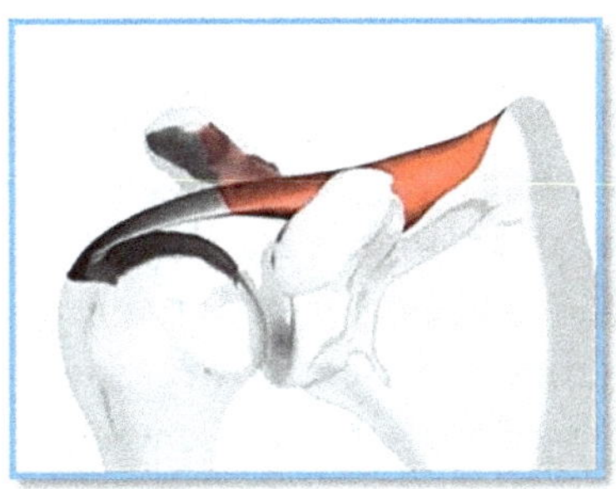

Your rotator cuff is extremely important to the body because it offers extraordinary range of motion. The rotator cuff is a group of tendons and muscles that sits in the shoulders and connects the upper arm to the shoulder blade.

If your rotator cuff is injured, you'll notice it almost instantly. For example, you won't be able to throw a ball overhead or pick up something off a shelf. Because your rotator cuff muscles are surrounded by bones, the interior pressure of your shoulder socket will increase if your rotator cuff becomes injured.

This will cause the muscle tissue to start to fray, since it will stop receiving a lot of blood. By getting a massage, you'll increase blood flow to your rotator cuff muscles, thus helping them heal.

Muscle Sprains and Strains

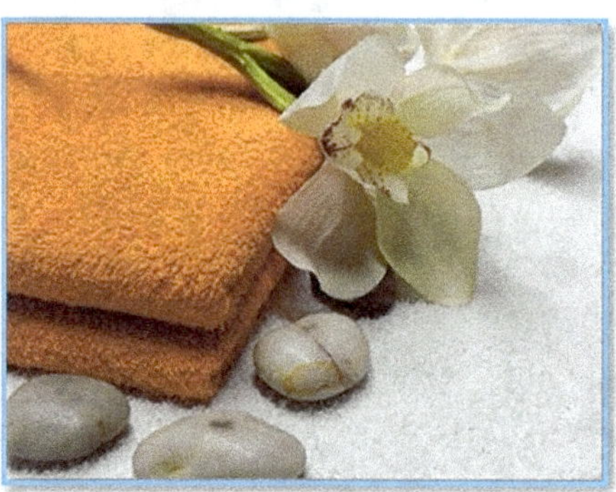

Massage therapy is a great way to efficiently treat muscle sprains and strains. This comes as no surprise considering that the massage therapist will spend all of their time during a session working on your soft tissues. Following a strain or a sprain, you will have to avoid engaging physical activity for several weeks, but thanks to massage therapy, you will fully recover after those weeks.

Myofascial Pain Syndrome

Myofascial pain syndrome is quite different from the muscle soreness you may feel after a challenging workout. One of the best ways to relieve myofascial pain is to get either a deep-tissue or a hot-stone massage.

It's worth noting that this syndrome is known to raise the risk of insomnia, depression, and anxiety. Thankfully, getting a massage suitable for relieving the symptoms of myofascial pain syndrome will help reduce these symptoms as well.

Effective Types of Massage for Myofascial Syndrome

Deep-tissue massage targets knots and helps release chronic tension by using stroking techniques against the grains of the muscles. Placing deep pressure on the fascia—the protective layer that surrounds bones, muscles, and joints—deep-tissue massage may feel uncomfortable during the session but provides lasting long-term benefits for the condition.

Hot-stone massage helps reach deeper layers of the muscles to reduce myofascial pain while at the same time increasing relaxation and reducing stress. The warm stones work to improve blood circulation and offer a sedative effect that helps relieve chronic pain.

Cancer

Massage therapy not only helps with pain related to cancer and treatments but it also helps fight the stress and anxiety associated with cancer diagnosis. On top of that, it will also help manage treatment side effects such as fatigue and nausea.

HIV

Massage therapy can help people suffering from HIV primarily by strengthening their immune system, thus helping them fight the disease. Additionally, it can help relieve certain HIV/AIDS symptoms, such as inflammation, body tension, cramps, and muscle spasms.

Sports Injuries

If a damaged muscle is massaged right away, there is a high chance of an extremely fast recovery. If you're an athlete and have suffered an injury but want to get back to working out quickly, then you should make sure to visit a massage therapist or a physical therapist as soon as possible. Massages are a great way to recover from sports injuries.

Carpal Tunnel Syndrome

If you experience numbness, tingling, or pain in your hands and wrists, then you might be suffering from carpal tunnel syndrome.

This syndrome usually affects the individual's dominant hand, which can negatively affect your movement.

Getting a massage tailored to fixing your problems with carpal tunnel syndrome will greatly reduce the symptoms associated with this condition.

Massage Is a Low-Risk Treatment

Massage has no side effects; it is a noninvasive low-risk treatment option for many conditions and general wellness.

Massage is also an excellent preventative measure. As an excellent tool in support of stress, it ensures that chronic stress does not cause the many chronic conditions it is associated with, and it supports your overall wellness and therefore quality of life.

Does Massage Hurt?

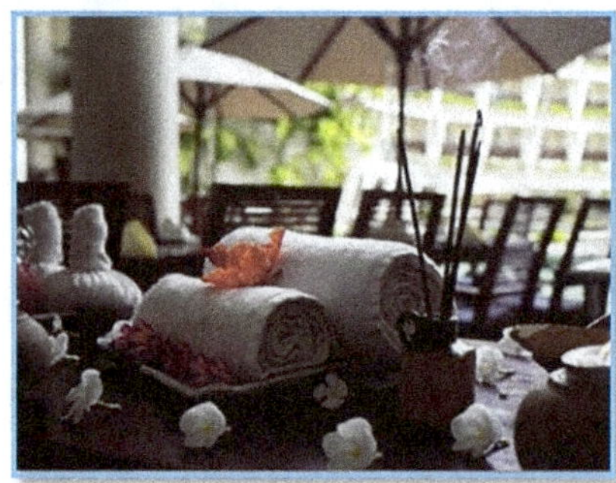

Normally, massage should not hurt, though this can depend on the condition being treated—with some discomfort being normal and a part of enjoying long-term relief and benefits.

Some people may experience some discomfort following their first or second session, but overall, the purpose of massage is for it to feel good during and make you feel better after a session.

If the typical relaxation massage hurts, it is important to tell the therapist performing it immediately; it is likely just a matter of applying less pressure.

Remember that the massage is for you and should be a pleasant experience.

Conditions Where Massage Is Not Advised

Most people can benefit from massage, but it is not appropriate if you have/are any of the following:

- Burns
- Healing wounds
- Taking blood-thinning medication or bleeding disorder
- Deep vein thrombosis
- Fractures
- Severe osteoporosis
- Severe thrombocytopenia
- Under the influence of drugs or alcohol

As a client, always advise your massage therapist the health conditions you may have, and likewise, they are always supposed to ask you of any medical conditions you might have.

Tips for Finding a Good Massage Therapist

Finding a good massage therapist is really important if you want to truly experience all the health benefits that you can gain from massage therapy. If you've never gotten a massage before, know that you won't be able to recognize a good therapist from a bad one simply by judging how your session went.

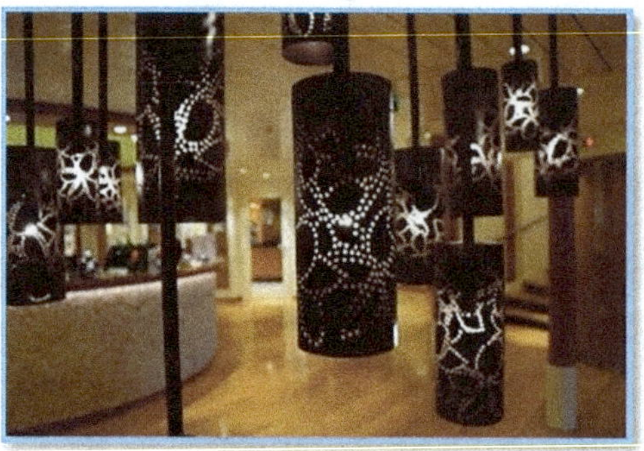

First and foremost, they should be licensed and certified in the state where they practice.

Massage is not just random kneading of the body but requires education and a comprehensive understanding of the human body, anatomy, and pressure points.

Knowledgeable and experienced massage therapists know exactly what to do and where and how to apply pressure to yield the best results.

Expert massage therapists also understand the connection between certain conditions and massage. For example, if you are pregnant, the massage therapist will use specific techniques to ensure your health and safety, as not all massage forms are appropriate for pregnant women. Well-trained therapists also understand how massage affects various medical conditions and injuries.

To make sure you're getting the real deal, you should check if the massage therapist you're about to book a session with is certified and licensed.

Reputable massage therapists are found in:

- Spas
- Health and fitness centers
- Massage clinics
- Hospitals
- Physical therapy centers
- Clinics
- Massage schools
- In-home services

For example, you can go on line to the AMTA, better known as the American Massage Therapy Association, at www.amtamassage. org and click on "Find a Massage Therapist." Then type in your city and zip code, and there you will find massage therapists in your area, complete with the services they offer and their contact information.

Final Thoughts

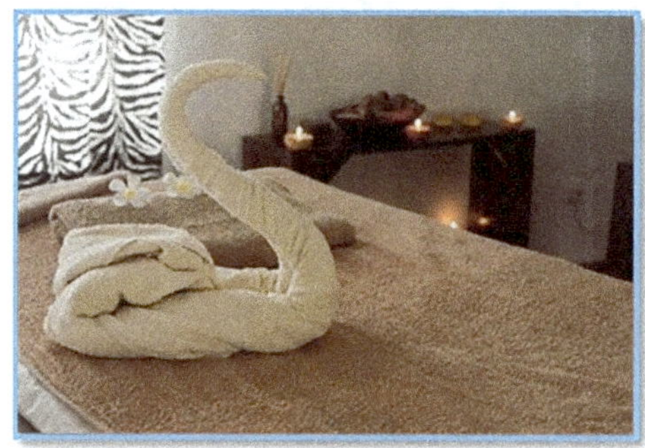

Massage therapy is used to manipulate your soft body tissues with the goal of improving your overall health. There are many different massage techniques, such as Swedish massage, shiatsu, deep-tissue massage, hot-stone massage, reflexology, aromatherapy massage, geriatric massage, and sports massage.

All of these different techniques offer varying health benefits.

Some of the most notable general health benefits of massages include relaxation, improved blood circulation, lower blood pressure, pain relief, depression management, enhanced mood, improved heart health, lower stress levels, anger management, better sleep, and a general boost in overall wellness of mind, body, and spirit.

Massage also helps in managing various chronic and acute medical ailments, along with pain conditions to speed up recovery and improve well-being.

With all of the health benefits it provides, massage therapy is considered to be one of the best forms of alternative medicine. It really can improve your quality of life, general health, and general wellness.

As a final note, it is very important to drink water after a massage. How much water should you drink after a massage? Usually, it is recommended that you drink six to eight glasses of water a day; however, after receiving a massage, it is advisable to increase it to ten glasses of water. You don't have to drink ten glasses of water all at once; you can space it out. For example, you can have two glasses of water in the morning with breakfast, two glasses of water before lunch, two glasses of water with lunch, two glasses of water with an afternoon snack, and two glasses of water with dinner. Why is it so important to drink water after a massage? It is so important to drink water after a massage because water helps flush all the toxins and lactic acids that have built up in the muscles caused by tension and stress. What will happen if you don't drink water after a massage? What will happen is that all the toxins and lactic acids will form back on the muscles causing you to feel bad. Such as feeling achy, sore, and nauseous. Almost like having flu-like symptoms. So if you start to feel this way, please increase your water intake; you will feel so much better!

I hope this book will serve your purpose well as you continue your journey on living a happy, healthy, and balanced life with massage therapy.

Acknowledgments

With special thanks to the following:

- My family and friends, thank you for your love and support over the years.
- All of the staff at the Atlanta School of Massage, thank you for teaching me how to become a successful massage therapist for twenty-one years.
- Dr. Goulburne and his staff, thank you so much for healing my back when I injured it.

References

1.   The psychological effects and benefits of sports massage (https://www.onsiteplus.com/benefits-sports-massage/)

2.   Benefits of Swedish Massage (https://www.massage2book.com/top-10-health-benefits-of-massage-therapies/top-10-health-benefits-of-Swedish-Massage/top-10-Swedish-Massage-benefits.html)

3.   Compression (www.physio.co.uk/treatments/massage/our-massage-techniques/compression.php

4.   Contraindications And Cautions For Deep Bodywork - Robert Schleip, Til Luchau and John Schewe. 8th edition, April 2018 (advanced-trainings.com/contraindications/)

5.   Precautions (https://www.encyclopedia.com/medicine/encyclopedias-almanacs-transcripts-and-maps/geriatric-massage)

6.   Contraindications of Lymph Massage (www.massage-mag.com/an-overview-of-manual-lymphatic-drainage-for-lymph)

7.   Contraindications of Pregnancy Massage (americanpregnancy.org/pregnancy.org/pregnancy-health/prenatal- massage/)

8.   Contraindications (www.reikiactivo.com/en/reiki/others/contraindications)

9.   Contraindications (shiatsu-london.net/contraindications.html)

10. Contraindications of Sports Massage (www.mesportsmassage.co.uk)

11. Contraindications of Swedish Massage (www.massagenow. com/contraindications/)

12. Contraindications of Therapeutic Touch (www.syrian-clinic.com/med/en/ProfModalities/Therapeutic Touch. html)

13. Cross Fiber (www.aglowbodyandskinspa.com/all-you-need-to- know-about-cross-Fibre-friction/)

14. Friction Strokes (www.massageprocedures.com/tech-niques- procedures/swedish-massage/friction)

15. Founders of Pregnancy Massage and History of It (paul-simpsonlmt.com/Pregnancy/Historyof PregnancyMassage. html)

16. Founder of Massage (www.sportsmassageinc.com/About-Jack- Meagher.htm)

17. Founders of Therapeutic Touch and What It Is (pennstate-hersey.adam.com/content.aspx?)

18. History of Aromatherapy Massage (www.aromatherapy. com/history.html)

19. History of Deep-Tissue Massage (www.leaf.tv/feel-good/ wellness/)

20. History of Lymph Massage (www.vodderschool.com/ manual_lymph_drainage_history)

21. History of Reflexology (en.wikipedia.org/wiki/Reflexology What is Zone Therapy?) (www.reflexheal.com)

22. History of Shiatsu Massage (www.shiatsusociety.org/ treatments/about-shiatsu)

23. History of Sports Massage (www.massagemag.com/a-brief- history-of-Sports-massage-25854/)

24. History of Swedish Massage (www.gamemassage.weebly. com/history-of-massage.html)

25. How Does Aromatherapy Work? (www.edu/health/ medical/altmed/treatment/aromatherapy

26. Jostling (www.books.google.com)

27. What Are the Benefits of Aromatherapy and Caution Using E. Oils (www.organicfacts.net/essential -oils-wrinkles.html)

28. What Are the Benefits of Geriatric Massage? (www.encyclopedia.com/medicine/encyclopedias-almanancs- transcripts -and-maps)
29. What Are the Benefits of a Hot-Stone Massage? (www.verywell.com/hot-stone-massage-89737)
30. What Are the Benefits of Reflexology? (naturallysavvy.com/care/10-health-benefits-of-reflexology)
31. What Are the Benefits of Shiatsu Massage (www.centerpointmn.com/the-benefits-of-shiatsu-massage/)
32. What Are the Benefits of Therapeutic Touch? (www.unh.edu/health/ohep/practices/therapeutic-touch)
33. What Are the Contraindications of Aromatherapy? (www.allthingszen.com/aromatherapy.php)
34. What Are the Contraindications of Hot-Stone Massage? (www.tranquiltouchmassage.com/CONTRAINDICATIONS)
35. What Are the Contraindications of Reflexology? (www.takingcharge.cshumm.edu/explore-healing- practices/reflexology/are-there-times-when-i-shoudn't-have- reflexology?)
36. What Is Aromatherapy? (www.thearomablog.com/aromatherapy- orgins-and-background)
37. What Is Aromatherapy Used For? (www.webmd.com> Healthand Balance>Stress Management)
38. What Is Deep-Tissue Massage and the Benefits of It (www.verywell.com/deep-tissue-massage-89738)
39. What Is Geriatric Massage? (www.encyclopedia.com/medicine/encylopedias-almanancs- transcripts-and-maps)
40. What Is Lymph Massage? (goodspaguide.co.uk/features/lymphatic- drainage-massage)
41. What Is Pregnancy Massage and Benefits of It (americanpregnancy.org/pregnancy.org/pregnancy-health/prenatal- massage/)
42. What Is Reflexology? (www.dr.weil.com/health- wellness/balanced-living/wellness-therapies/reflexology/)
43. What Is Shiatsu Massage (www.amcollege.edu/blog/health-benefits-of-shiatsu-massage therapy)

44. What Is a Sports Massage? (wikipedia.org/wiki/Myofacial-trigger_point)

45. What Is the History of Hot-Stone Massage? (www.hahana.comon/history-of-stone-massage)

46. What Is Reiki and Benefits of It (www.manitouwellness.com/what- we-do-/7-health-benefits-of-reiki/)

47. Where Did Geriatric Massage Originate From? (www.encyclopedia.com/medicine/encyclopedias-almanancs-transcripts-and-maps)

48. Where Did Lymph Massage Originate From? (en.wikipedia.org/wiki/Manual_lymphatic_drainage)

49. Where Did Sports Massage Originate From? (www.massagetutor.com/wp-content/uploads/2015/03/Sports-Massage-History.pdf)

50. Where Did Reiki Originate From? (en.wikipedia.org/wiki/Reiki History of Reiki (www.thethirstysoul.com/reiki/history-of-reiki/)

51. Where Did Pregnancy Massage Originate From? (www.zenmindbody.co.uk/pregnancy-massage/)

52. Where Did Therapeutic Touch Originate From (www.westernschools.com/portals/11/html/N1543/miWRpi_files/…/Chap9.html)

Contact Information

If you loved my book and want to write a short review about it you can contact me at www.holisiticcareandmassage.com/contact and Facebook.com/holisticcareandmassage.com/contact Thank you! Your reviews are greatly appreciated!

About the Author

Katherine Smith is originally from Atlanta, Georgia, where she attended the Atlanta School of Massage and graduated in 1996. Upon graduating, she was accepted as a member of the American Massage Association since 1997. She is currently retired and likes to travel with her husband, relax on the beach, and enjoy writing articles and blogs about massage therapy.

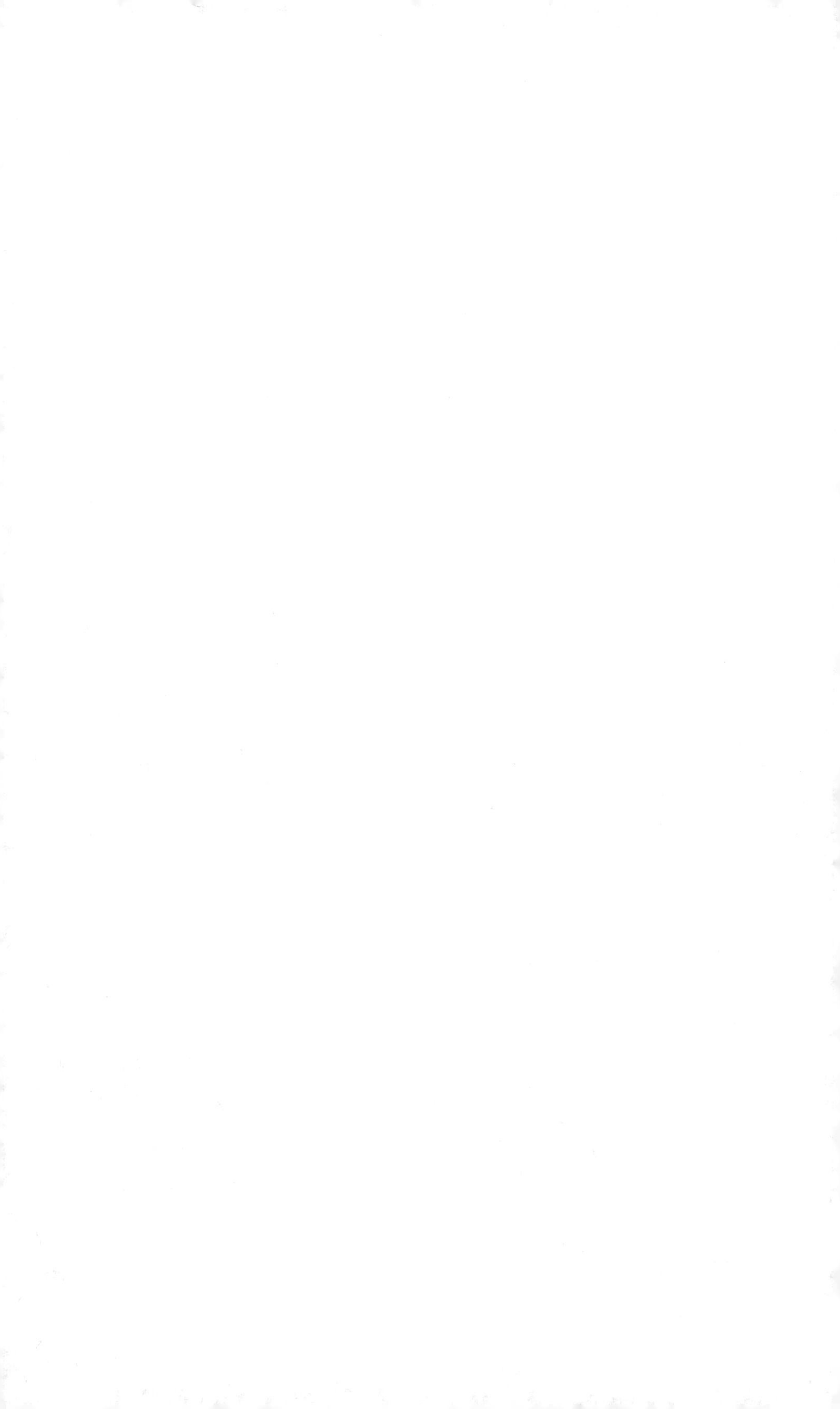